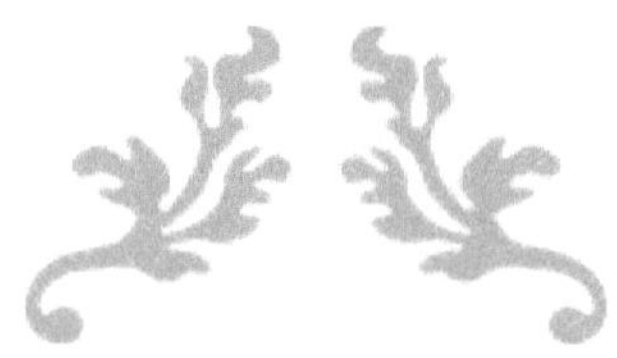

SMOOTHIES FOR HEALTHY HAIR AND SKIN

Quick Guide

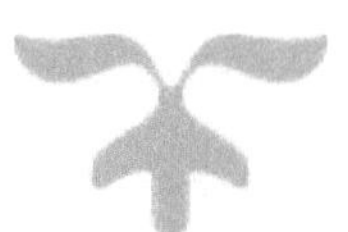

BY ZENA XENAE

Title ID: **7536039**
ISBN-13: **978-1976057571**

This book is dedicated to the loving memory of my cousin, Pamela Arlyce Moorman A.K.A "Pam". My biggest fan and cheerleader. I love you to the heavens and back!

Contents

Introduction

 In 2014, I was diagnosed with breast cancer after numerous surgeries and chemo I completed my cancer treatments in August of 2015. It was a depressing time. The chemo took its toll on my skin and my hair leaving me completely bald. I met with the nutritionist in the oncology center and she provided me with a list of foods and vegetables that would be beneficial in getting me feeling back to normal. I realized there was no way for me to consume all the items on the list daily, so I started making smoothies. I blended them together to get better results, within 16 months, I went from bald to having armpit length thick hair. My skin was radiant. The other tips and tricks on how I grew my hair back so fast, can be found in my book "Chemo Curls."

The purpose of this book is to give you the recipes to some of the most delicious and nutritious smoothies out there green or not. Designed to provide you with the necessary nutrients to grow strong, healthy hair, while providing you with radiant glowing skin. The rest of your body will also benefit from your consumption of these delicious smoothies. Yes, you could take hair, skin, and nail vitamins, but it is best coming from the most natural source. And because you are making it you will know exactly what's going into your body.

In addition to drinking smoothies it is imperative that you develop and stick to a good hair and skin care regimen. Try to avoid products with sulfates, parabens, and mineral oil. Minimize heat usage on your hair and exercise protective styling. Remember to wear sun screen when outdoors and keep your skin moisturized. This will give you optimal results.

The recipes in this book have been tried by and me and have given me great results. Don't be afraid to experiment and try different flavor combinations that you normally would not try. Life is too short to taste the same every day. You are on your way to looking and feeling better every day. Enjoy!

Why drink smoothies?

Smoothies are a great way to nourish your bodies from the Inside Out. Drinking your fruit and vegetables assures that you are getting your daily supply of vitamins and nutrients without the use of supplements. This allows you to pick all the fruits and vegetables you like, as well as the ones that you otherwise would skip. Blending them gives them flavor, while giving you all the necessary nutrients to acquire healthier hair and radiant skin.

Drinking smoothies also has other health benefits such as detoxing your body, boosting your immune system, preventing diabetes, weight loss, improved digestion and some say they may decrease your risk of cancer.

The key to a great smoothie is to make sure you are choosing healthy organic ingredients. Most smoothies will consist of at least 1 cup of leafy greens, 1 cup of liquid and 2 cups of fruit. This combination will give you the best nutritional blend and flavor.

The other important thing is to make sure you have invested in a good, high power blender. Nothing ruins a smoothie quicker than it not being blended correctly. As a rule, blend your greens and liquid together, then add your frozen fruits. I personally use the Ninja IQ of all the ones I have tried I love this one the most. Of course, there are others out there that work just as well, this is just my favorite.

Lastly, don't forget to dress up your smoothie. Adding nuts, granola, yogurt, and fresh fruit your smoothie, packs an additional punch of nutrition and flavor. Not to mention you can get creative with your garnishes making that smoothie appealing to the eye and seemingly more delicious!

Commonly used Ingredients in smoothies and their benefits

Here are a few ingredients you can use in a Smoothie:

- Fruits: Berries, strawberries blueberries, raspberries, bananas, melons, apples pears, oranges, cherries, pineapples, kiwi, etc.
- Peanut butter, almond butter
- Sweetener-Honey, stevia, maple syrup, organic coconut sugar. Molasses.
- Ground flax seeds, hemp, maca powder, chia seeds, cocoa powder, wheatgrass
- Milk (almond, coconut, cashew, rice, etc.) I don't prefer cow's milk because of possible hormones and steroids.
- Veggies- kale, spinach, lettuce, carrots, celery, cucumber, sweet potato, squash, etc.
- Water-Filtered or spring
- Juices-fresh organic 100% fruit juice

List of a few smoothie ingredients and how they aid in the health of your skin and hair

Apple Cider Vinegar- Super food of the super foods, this has so many benefits it's hard to name all of them. Lowers blood pressure, improve diabetes, supports weight loss, helps balance PH levels in skin.

Avocado-Often referred to as a superfood, Avocado is high in healthy fats. The fat in them allows you to better absorb your nutrients from plant foods. Mixing your avocado with other veggies can increase the amount of antioxidants you take in, leading to ageless skin.

Bananas -Provides the hair natural oils, silica which will help soften and moisten your hair making it more manageable. It aids in preventing split ends

Blueberries-Loaded with antioxidants, protects skin from premature aging

Carrots-Contains Vitamin A needed to help the body produce Sebum which is needed for the health of the scalp.

Chia Seeds-contains omega-3 fatty acids, protein, fiber antioxidants and calcium. They are also an energy booster.

Cucumber- contains anti-inflammatory agents, diuretic helps with water retention.

Coconut-has healthy fats, vitamin E and K. Natural nutrients to aid in the growth of the hair.

Dragon Fruit- has a number of phytonutrients, low sugar content. Rich in antioxidants and vitamin B and C. Fights signs of aging and acne.

Greek Yogurt- loaded with B5 to aid in the circulation of blood to the scalp. It has double the amount of protein as regular yogurt with fewer carbohydrates and sugar. Your hair is made of protein, including more Greek yogurt in your diet will prevent hair loss.

Guava-packed with vitamin C, folic acid, potassium, and fiber. Guava protects your hair from breaking.

Honey-considered a complexion boost has been used for centuries by women for it's beauty enhancing properties. Helps combat dry hair.

Kale-has many beneficial properties loaded with iron, antioxidants, vitamin A and K, keeps hair moisturized. It keeps skin looking great and helps reverse skin damage. It is said to help prevent cancer as it rids the body of toxins.

Kiwi-packed with vitamin A and E, will assist in the elimination of free radicals.

Lemons-good source of vitamin C

Melons-cantaloupe, watermelon, honeydew melon are a great source of vitamin C. Vitamin C is the most effective nutrient to help strengthen and grow hair. It also helps builds collagen essential to hair and skin health.

Mustard greens– aids in strong healthy hair great source of vitamin C and E contains beta- carotene and folate.

Pineapple-softens skin high in vitamin C, has Amino Acids which aid in skin repair.

Raspberries-for radiant skin they contain anthocyanins, which help add color to the berry as well as your skin. They contain vitamin C and Carotene, which help to fight damage caused by free radicals.

Romaine lettuce-has lots of hair nutrient properties, beta carotene, vitamin C Folate and Iron

Spinach- provides nutrients to the hair follicles, contains iron which helps carry oxygen to the hair. It helps dry brittle hair.

Strawberries- contains Biotin which aids in the growth of hair. Great for skin contains anti-aging properties, may help fight carcinogens.

Sweet Potato-contains beta-carotene, A. B6, C, D and calcium, considered a hair growth booster and combats many deficiencies your hair may have, dull, lifeless and dry.

Squash can improve the health of your hair, skin and nails. High in vitamin A, B, C and E.

A grocery list has been provided in the back of book for your convenience.

Smoothie Order for a Perfect Blend

Always pack your blender from the softest to the hardest.

8

TIP! Add only half the amount of liquid the recipe calls for first, then check

 your consistency before adding remaining Ingredients. This will prevent mishaps!

6 Frozen Fruit or Ice

5 Fresh fruits, nuts, flaxseeds

4 Soft Ingredients – yogurt, nut butters

3 Leafy Greens

2 Powders

1 Liquid first, milk, juices, water. Save half to add in

 last.

SMOOTHIE RECIPES

This chapter contains all my favorite smoothie recipes. The recipes marked as an author favorite are on the top of my list.

Hopefully you will find your favorite combo that you will love or make it your own. You will find that these recipes are formulated with ingredients to target hair growth and will create ageless glowing skin. These smoothie recipes will deliver nutrients, vitamins and some cancer fighting agents.

Green Tea and Pineapple Smoothie

2 servings

Ingredients

2 cups of fresh pineapple (peeled and chopped)

1 cup green tea made from loose leaves

1 tsp honey

½ inch of fresh ginger, peeled and chopped

1 cup of ice

1 slice of pineapple for garnish

Directions

Combine all ingredients in a blender and process until smooth

Garnish with a slice of pineapple

Caribbean Green Smoothie

Serves 2

Ingredients

1 apple

1 sliced banana

12 white grapes

1 cup kale

1 cup fresh pineapple

½ cup spring or filtered water

½ lemon peeled

Lemon or lime slice for garnish

2-3 cubes of ice

Directions

Place all ingredients in blender blend until smooth. Garnish with lemon or lime.

The Honey I Won't Be Home Tonight Smoothie

Serves 2

Ingredients t

2 cups chopped yellow watermelon

1 cup white seedless grapes

½ cup frozen pineapple chunks

1 sliced banana

1 cup coconut water

1-2 Ice cubes

Directions

Place all ingredients in blender blend until smooth. Garnish with watermelon slice or pineapple.

Banana and Cantaloupe Smoothie

Author Favorite

1-2 servings

Ingredients

1 large banana, sliced and frozen
1 cup cantaloupe, seeded and coarsely chopped
1 cup almond Milk
1 vanilla bean (seeds only)
1 teaspoon of honey or stevia

3-4 cubes of ice

Directions

Place all ingredients in a blender or with ice closest to blade blend until smooth. Garnish as desired.

Cucumber Honeydew Smoothie

1-2 servings

Ingredients

1 1/2 cup cucumber, unpeeled, chopped
(most nutrients are in the peel)
1 1/2 cup honeydew melon, chopped
1 cup plain non-fat yoghurt with probiotic bacteria
1 fresh mint, chopped
1 tsp fresh lemon juice
1 cup crushed ice

<u>Garnish</u>
Lemon wedges
Fresh mint leaves

Directions

Place all ingredients in blender, blend to desired consistency.

Garnish with lemon and mint

Coconut Pear Smoothie

1-2 servings

Ingredients

½ cup of almond Milk
½ cup of coconut water or coconut milk
1 medium pear
1 small handful of kale –
½ teaspoon coconut extract
4 or 5 ice cubes

<u>Garnish</u>

Coconut flakes

Directions

Combine all ingredients into blender and blend until smooth.

Garnish with coconut flakes

Cherry Nut Smoothie

Serves 1-2

Ingredients

1-cup kale

½ frozen banana

1 1/2 cups frozen dark sweet cherries

2 tablespoons organic almond butter

1/2-cup almond milk

¼ tsp vanilla extract or 3 drops vanilla crème stevia

2-3 ice cubes

<u>Garnish</u>

Dannon Cherry Cheesecake Mouse

Cherry

Chocolate Banana Nut granola

Directions

Place all ingredients into blender, blend until smooth. Garnish with Dannon Greek Mousse Cherry Cheesecake Yogurt, sprinkle with chocolate banana nut granola and top with a cherry!

Berry Banana Smoothie

Targets skin and hair!

Serves 1-2

Ingredients

1-cup spinach

1.5 cups of frozen mixed berries

1 banana sliced

2 tsp rolled oats

1-cup almond milk or coconut milk

3-4 cubes of ice

<u>Garnish</u>

coconut flakes

Directions

Blend all ingredients except coconut flakes until smooth. Garnish with coconut flakes.

Mean Green Mango Smoothie

Serves 1-2

18

Ingredients

½ cup kale

½ cup spinach frozen

1.5 cup mango

¼ vanilla Greek Yogurt

1 cup coconut water

½ apple

3-4 cubes of ice

<u>Garnish</u>

Slice of lemon

Directions

Blend until smooth. Garnish with a slice of lemon.

Banana Pineapple Kale Smoothie

Serves 1-2

19

Ingredients

2 cups kale

¼ cup pineapple

¾ almond milk

1 banana

¼ Greek yogurt

1 tsp honey

Directions

Blend until creamy, garnish as desired.

Strawberry Banana Smoothie

serves 1-2

20

Ingredients

1 cup strawberries

1 banana

¼ cup granola

1 cup Greek yogurt

1 tsp chia seeds

3-4 cubes of ice

Directions

Blend until smooth, garnish as desired.

Blueberry Mango Smoothie

Serves 1-2

Ingredients

1 cup blueberries

1 ½ mango

½ avocado

1 tsp honey

1 tsp chia seeds

½ pear sliced

1 ½ cups coconut water

2-3 cubes of ice

Directions

Blend until smooth, garnish as desired.

Chocolate Delight Smoothie

Serves 1-2

22

Ingredients

1 cup spinach

1 banana

3 tsp cocoa powder

½ tsp vanilla stevia liquid

1 tsp chia seeds

½ cup chocolate yogurt

Garnish

Vanilla Greek yogurt

Granola

Directions

Place all ingredients in blender except Vanilla yogurt, blend until smooth. Garnish with Vanilla Greek Yogurt and granola. Carefully lay mixture into glass into layers mixing chocolate with the vanilla yogurt. Use toothpick or straw to create lines.

Mango Berry Smoothie

Serves 1-2

Ingredients

½ cup raspberries

1 cup frozen strawberries

1 cup mango

¼ cup mango juice

½ cup Vanilla Greek yogurt

3-4 cubes of Ice

Directions

Blend until smooth and creamy

Garnish with a strawberry and slice of mango.

Merry Berry Smoothie

Serves 1-2

Ingredients

1 cup Raspberries

1 cup Blueberries

1 cup Strawberries

½ cup cherries

1 2/2 guava juice

2-3 cubes of ice

<u>Garnish</u>

Save a few berries for garnish

Directions

Blend until smooth

Garnish with berries

Summer Breeze Smoothie

Serve 1-2

Ingredients

2 kiwis

1½ cup seedless grapes

1 ½ cups strawberries

1 cup watermelon seedless

½ cup mango

1 cup coconut water

2-3 ice cubes

Directions

Blend until smooth and creamy, garnish as desired.

Peachy Green Smoothie

Serves 1-2

26

Ingredients

1 cup spinach

1 cup Blueberries

I cup peaches

½ peach yogurt

1 cup guava juice

2-3 ice cubes

Directions

Blend until smooth and creamy, garnish as desired.

The Greenery Smoothie

Serves 1

Ingredients

2 slices of watermelon

Few leaves of fresh mint

½ bag of fresh baby spinach

½ cup mango frozen

½ avocado

½ cucumber

2 tsp Greek yogurt plain

1 ½ cups apple juice

1 tsp stevia optional

Directions

Put the spinach and 1 cup of apple juice in blender. Blend the spinach down then add all remaining ingredients blend till smooth.

Inside Out

Banana Berry Spinach Smoothie

Serves 1-2

Ingredients

½ cup spinach

1 banana

1 cup frozen mixed berries

1 tsp chia seeds

1 tsp flaxseeds

½ cup Almond Milk

1 tsp liquid vitamin B complex (optional) gives an extra boost

3-4 Ice cubes

Directions

Blend all ingredients until smooth and creamy

Inside Out

Red Berry Apple Smoothie

Serves 1-2

Ingredients

1 apple

½ cup frozen raspberry

½ cup frozen strawberries

½ frozen sweet cherries

1 cup red grapes

½ cup kale

½ tsp flax seeds

½ chia seeds

1 cup coconut water or ¼ of your blender container whichever is less

3-4 ice cups

<u>Garnish</u>

 Greek yogurt, berries, and granola

Directions

Place all ingredients in blender, except yogurt and granola save some berries for garnish.

Garnish with Greek yogurt, berries, and granola.

Triple Berry Boost Smoothie

Serves 1-2

Ingredients

1 cup mixed frozen berries

½ cup sweet dark cherries

½ cup pineapple

½ apple

1 tsp milled flaxseeds

1 tsp lemon juice

1 tsp liquid B Complex

1 cup pineapple coconut water

2-3 ice cups

Blend all ingredients together until smooth

<u>Garnish</u>

Vanilla yogurt and berries.

Directions

Place all items in blender except yogurt, save some berries for your garnish blend until smooth.

Inside Out

Yellow Sunday Morning Smoothie

Serves 1-2

Ingredients

1 Banana

1 yellow squash include peel

1 cup pineapple

1 apple

1 navel orange

½ lemon include peel

½ tsp organic coconut sugar

3-4 cups of ice

½ cup coconut water

<u>Garnish</u>

Slice of lemon

Granola

Directions

Blend all ingredients until smooth and creamy

Garnish with lemon slice and granola

Tropical Kale Smoothie

Serves 1-2

Ingredients

2 cups kale

1 cup pineapple

1 cup mango

1 cup coconut chunks

I cup mango juice

1 tsp flaxseed

2 tbsp chia seeds or hemp seeds

1 tsp organic honey

<u>Garnish</u>

Pineapple slice

Coconut flakes

1 strawberry

Directions

Blend the kale with the mango juice then add frozen fruit and the rest of ingredients. Garnish with pineapple slice, strawberry, and mango.

Fuchsia Fruit Smoothie

Serves 1-2

Ingredients

1 cup of dragon fruit (red) or *Pitaya puree

1 frozen banana

1 cup coconut water

1 tsp ginger

½ cup mango

2-3 ice cubes

Directions

Blend all ingredients in a blender until smooth. Pour into glass. Garnish as desired.

*Note if you cannot find dragon fruit at your grocery store, you can find the organic Pitaya plus packs online at www.pitayaplus.com

Pumpkin Pie Smooth

Serves 1 -2

Ingredients

½ cup pumpkin puree

4 oz. Greek yogurt

½ cup water

1/4 avocado

2 TBSP ground flaxseed

½ tsp pumpkin pie spice

Directions

Place all ingredients in blender, blend until smooth and creamy. Garnish with a cinnamon stick and pumpkin spice.

Mango Surprise Smoothie

Serves 1

Ingredients

¼ cup mango cubes

¼ cup mashed ripe avocado

½ cup mango juice

¼ cup Greek Vanilla yogurt

1 tsp. fresh lime juice

1 tbsp. Stevia (optional)

6 ice cubes

Directions

Combine all the ingredients into the blender, process until smooth. Garnish with a slice of mango and a strawberry. **Note whenever using ice in a recipe always check consistency before adding more.

Green Wonder Smoothie

Serves 2

Ingredients

1 ¼ cup frozen kale

1 ¼ cup frozen mango

2 med celery stalks chopped

1 cup frozen orange juice

¼ cup parsley chopped

a few mint leaves (save some for garnish)

Directions

Place all items in blender, blend until smooth. Garnish with mint. You may have to repeat the blend cycle to get exact smoothness.

Gingered Cantaloupe Smoothie

Serves 2

Ingredients

2 cups cantaloupe

½ grated ginger

3 tsp. stevia

3-4 cubes of Ice

Directions

Combine all ingredients into blender and blend until smooth Serve in half of cantaloupe. Garnish with mint.

Healthy High C Smoothie

Serves 1

Ingredients

1 cup frozen chopped kale

2 kiwis, peeled and chopped

½ cup fresh orange juice

¼ cup cilantro

1 stalk of celery chopped

3-4 ice cubes

Directions

Place all ingredients in blender, blend until smooth.

Carrot Cake Smoothie

Serves 1

Ingredients

½ cup unsweetened carrot juice

1 scoop Vanilla Greek yogurt

2 Tbsp toasted wheat germ

1 Tbsp cream cheese softened

¼ tsp ground cinnamon

2-4 ice cubes

1 tsp stevia

Directions

Place all ingredients in blender and blend until smooth

Inside Out

Winter Greens Smoothie

Serves 2

40

Ingredients

¼ cup carrot juice

½ cup orange

1 cup spinach

1 cup frozen kale

banana sliced and peeled

1 apple sliced

Directions

Place kale, spinach and orange juice in blender and blend until smooth. Add all remaining ingredients and blend well

Apricot Smoothie

Serves 2

Ingredients

12 pitted apricots

1 cup skim milk

¾ cup Greek yogurt Vanilla

½ tsp almond extract

Directions

Combine all ingredients in blender, blend until smooth.

Glam Life Smoothie

Targets skin with antioxidants!

Serves 2

Ingredients

¼ cup orange juice

½ cup Plain Greek yogurt

1 cup frozen mixed berries

1 cup frozen spinach

½ sliced frozen banana

6 baby carrots

Orange slice for garnish

Directions

Place yogurt and orange juice in blender blend until smooth then add the remaining ingredients. Garnish with slice of orange

Green King Smoothie

Serves 1

Ingredients

1 cup baby spinach

1 cup cucumber sliced

½ cup avocado halved and peeled

1 kiwi peeled and pitted

¼ cup Greek yogurt

½ cup pineapple coconut water

¼ mint leaves

Directions

Place all ingredients in blender and blend until smooth.

Banana Ginger Smoothie

Serves 2

Ingredients

1 banana sliced

¾ cup vanilla yogurt

1 tbsp honey

½ tsp grated ginger

Directions

Place all ingredients into blender and blend until smooth

Orange Dream

Author Favorite

Serves 1

Ingredients

1 navel orange

¼ cup vanilla yogurt

2 tbsp frozen orange juice concentrate

¼ tsp vanilla extract

4 ice cubes

Directions

Place all ingredients in blender with the ice closest to the blade blend to desired thickness.

Green Tea, Blueberry, and Banana

Antioxidant rich

Serves 1

Ingredients

¼ cup green tea

2 tsp honey

1 ½ cup frozen blueberries

1 banana

1/4 cup almond milk

Directions

Combine all ingredients into blender and blend until smooth

Orange Breakfast Smoothie

Serves 1

Ingredients

1 cup vanilla Greek yogurt

1 frozen banana sliced

½ cup orange juice

6 frozen strawberries

Directions

Place all ingredients in blender, blend to your desired consistency
check often during blend cycle

Tropical Pineapple Passion

Serves 1

Ingredients

1 cup Greek yogurt

1 cup crushed ice

1 whole pineapple

1 tsp organic honey

1 cup pineapple chucks (cut from pineapple)

2 tbsp. coconut rum (optional, but I know you were thinking it)

Garnish-1 pineapple ring, 1 cherry and coconut flakes

Directions

Slice tip off pineapple and use pineapple corer to remove inside of pineapple. Clean contents of pineapple so that the pineapple shell can be used as a cup.

Slice pineapple into chucks, place pineapple chunks and all remaining ingredients into blender blend until smooth. (add ice slowly and check consistency.) Garnish with pineapple, coconut flakes optional. Enjoy!

Strawberry-Kiwi Smoothie

Serves 4

Ingredients

1 ¼ cup chilled apple juice

1 frozen banana sliced

1 kiwi peeled and sliced

5 frozen strawberry

Directions

Combine all ingredients in blender, blend until smooth.

Banana Blueberry Smoothie

Serves 2

Ingredients

1 cup almond milk

½ cup frozen blueberries

½ sliced frozen banana

2 tsp stevia

1 tsp vanilla extract

Directions

Place all ingredients in blender and blend until smooth. Garnish with blueberries.

Tropical Papaya Perfection

Serves 1

51

Ingredients

1 papaya cut into chucks

1 cup Greek yogurt

1 navel orange sliced and peeled

½ cup pineapple

½ cup crushed ice

1 tsp coconut extract

1 tsp ground flaxseed

Directions

Place all ingredients in blender, blend until smooth and frosty.

Just Peachy

Serves 2

52

Ingredients

1 cup almond milk

2 tbsp low fat vanilla yogurt

½ cup frozen strawberries

½ cup frozen peaches

½ tsp powdered ginger

Directions

Combine all ingredients into blender, blend until smooth.

Apricot-Mango Madness

Serves 2

Ingredients

6 apricots peeled seeded and chopped

2 cups mangos peeled and chopped

1 cup almond milk

4 tsp fresh lemon juice

½ cup vanilla extract

4-6 ice cubes

Lemon zest- for garnish

Directions

Place all ingredients except lemon zest in blender (gradually add ice to check for consistency) blend until smooth. Garnish with lemon zest

Dreamy Melon Smoothie

Serves 2

Ingredients

2 cups chopped seedless watermelon

¼ almond milk

6-8 cubes of ice

Directions

Blend the watermelon and milk until smooth, slowly add in ice until it reaches your desired thickness

Morning Sunrise Smoothie

Serves 2

55

Ingredients

1 banana

1 cup apricot nectar chilled

8oz low fat peach yogurt

1 tbsp. frozen lemonade concentrate

½ cup club soda chilled

Directions

Combine all ingredients except club soda in blender blend until smooth. 'slowly stir in club soda, serve immediately.

Vanilla Berry Smoothie

Serves 2

Ingredients

½ cup frozen raspberries

½ cup frozen strawberries

¾ unsweetened pineapple juice

1 cup fat free vanilla yogurt

Directions

Combine the all ingredients blend until smooth.

Tutti Smoothie

Serves 2

57

Ingredient

½ cup mixed frozen berries'

½ cup crushed pineapple

½ cup plain Greek yogurt

½ sliced banana

½ cup orange juice

2-3 ice cubes

Directions

Combine all the ingredients blend until smooth.

Watermelon Papaya Smoothie

Serves 1

58

Ingredients

1 cup sliced seedless watermelon

2 papayas peeled

4 blueberries

4 mint leaves

Directions

Place all ingredients in blender except mint leaves and blueberries. Blend until smooth. Garnish with blueberries and mint leaves

.

Banana-Coconut Smoothie

Serves 1

Ingredients

1 cup almond milk (or milk of choice)

1 frozen banana

2 tbsps. unsweetened coconut

1 cup vanilla yogurt

Directions

Place all ingredients into blender fruit first, blend until smooth. Garnish as desired

Pineapple Berry Smoothie

Serves

Ingredients

½ cup blueberries

½ cup raspberries

½ frozen banana

¼ cup diced pineapple

2 tbsps. chia seeds

3 ice cubes

½ cup pomegranate juice

Directions

Place all items into blender fruit first blend until smooth. Garnish with a slice of pineapple

Strawberry Pomegranate Smoothie

Serves 1

Ingredients

¼ cup pomegranate juice

2 tsp organic honey

¾ cup frozen strawberries

2 tbsp plain fat free yogurt

1 tbsp flaxseeds

4 ice cubes

Directions

Mix all ingredients together in blender until it reaches desired consistency.

Blueberry Beet Almond Smoothie

Serves 2

62

Ingredients

½ cup carrot juice

½ cup frozen blueberries

½ cup raw beets peeled and grated

½ cup unsweetened apple sauce

½ cup unsalted almonds

6 ice cubes

½ tsp lime juice

Lemon slice for garnish

Dash of ginger

Directions Combine all ingredients in a blender and blend until smooth and creamy. Serve Immediately. Garnish with lemon.

Mango-Avocado Smoothie

Serves 1

Ingredients

½ fresh mango

1 cup fresh or frozen spinach

1 cup chilled coconut or almond milk (or lowfat milk

¼ avocado

3 tsp stevia

Directions

Place ingredients in a blender, blend until smooth. You can add or remove ice for desired thickness.

Almond, Blueberry, and Banana Smoothie

Hair Booster! This recipe may help with dry hair if consumed daily.

Serves 1

Ingredients

1 ½ cups unsweetened almond milk

¾ frozen banana

1 cup frozen blueberries

1 cup chopped kale

5 unsalted almonds

2 teaspoons organic honey

1 tsp granola for garnish

Directions

1. Whisk honey and almond milk together.

2. Place all fruit and kale into blender

3. Add remaining ingredients. (milk mixture) and blend until smooth.

4. Garnish with blueberries and granola

Orange Kale Smoothie

Serves 1

t

Ingredients

1 navel orange peeled

1 cup fresh kale

½ tsp Spirulina Powder

1 pinch ginger powder

1 cup orange juice

Directions

Place all ingredients in blender blend until smooth, may add ice to thicken.

Blueberry Mint Smoothie

Serves 2

Ingredients

2 cups frozen spinach

2 cups frozen blueberries

1 kiwi

3-4 large mint leaves (save some for garnish)

1 cup coconut water

1 cup ice

Directions

Place all ingredients in blender and blend until smooth, Garnish with mint leaves.

Green Pineapple Smoothie

Serves 2

Ingredients

1 ½ cups frozen spinach

1 ½ cups spinach

1 ½ cups pineapple

½ banana

½ cup almond milk

½ cup coconut water

2 -3 cubes of ice

Directions

Place all ingredients in blender blend until it reaches your desired consistency. Garnish with pineapple slice.

Minted Dew Smoothie

Serves 4

Ingredients

½ honeydew melon cut into chunks

½ cup coconut milk

6 mint leaves (save some for garnish)

½ tsp fresh lime juice

1 cup ice

1 tsp honey

Directions

Add all ingredients into blender fruit first, then fill with liquid ingredients. Serve in chilled glasses. Garnish with mint.

Grape Berry Smoothie

Serves 2

Ingredients

1 tsp chia seeds

1 cup seedless red grapes

½ cup blueberries

1 tsp flaxseed

½ cup coconut water

Directions

Place all ingredients into blender, blend until smooth. Garnish as desired.

Apple Pie Smoothie

Serves 2

Ingredients

2 large apples peeled and cored

1 frozen banana

1 cup ice

1 cup almond milk

½ cup Greek Yogurt

1 tsp ground cinnamon

Pinch of nutmeg

Pinch of ground ginger

1-2 tsp stevia

Directions

Place all ingredients in blender, blend until smooth, Garnish with cinnamon or cinnamon sticks

.

Tropical Turmeric Smoothie

Targets hair and skin improves circulation!

Serves 2-4

Ingredients

2 cups frozen kale

¼ cup cilantro

2 cups coconut water

2 cups chopped pineapple

1 cup chopped mango

½ cup lemon juice fresh squeezed

½ tsp ground turmeric

Directions

Blend kale, cilantro, and coconut, then add remaining ingredients blend again until smooth. Garnish as desired.

Coconut Papaya Smoothie

Serves 2

72

Ingredients

2 cups frozen spinach

2 cups unsweetened coconut water

1 navel orange peeled

1 cup of seeded chopped papaya

1 cup strawberries

Directions

Blend spinach and coconut water together, then add remaining ingredients and blend until smooth.

Radiant Cooler

Serves 2

Ingredients

2 cups spinach

2 cups chopped watermelon

1 sliced orange

1 cup strawberries

Directions

Blend the spinach and watermelon until smooth

Add the peaches and strawberries and blend until smooth

Pineapple Mojito

Serves 2

Ingredients

2 cups frozen kale

¼ cup fresh mint leaves

2 cups coconut water

3 cups chop pineapple

1 freshly squeezed lime

Directions

Place all ingredients in blender, blend until smooth. Garnish as desired

Glowing Berry

Serves 2

Ingredients

1 ½ cups frozen spinach

½ cup fresh mint leaves

2 cups unsweetened coconut water

2 cups blackberries

2 cups kiwi

Directions

Add in spinach, mint, and coconut water until smooth then add remaining ingredients and blend again until smooth.

Summer Glow

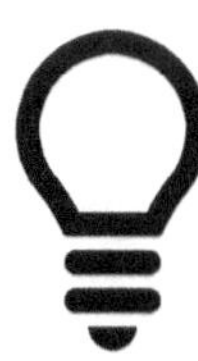

Target sun kissed skin!

Serves 2

Ingredients

2 cups collard greens

1 cup water

1 cup chopped cantaloupe

2 cups chopped mango

½ cup chopped carrots

½ chopped pineapple

Directions

Blend collards, water, and cantaloupe, then add in carrots, pineapple and blend until smooth.

Watermelon Banana Smoothie

Serves 2

Ingredients

1 1/2 cups fresh watermelon, cubed seeds removed

1 cup frozen strawberries

1/2 ripe banana chopped and frozen

½ cup unsweetened plain almond milk

1 lime, juiced

1 Tbsp. chia or hemp seeds

2-3 cubes ice as needed to thicken

Instructions

Place all ingredients in blender blend until smooth. Making sure to check consistency of melons as they liquefy causes more juice to release.

Strawberry Watermelon Smoothie

The high-water content in this smoothie makes an excellent skin hydrator!

Serves 1-2

ingredients

1 cup watermelon

1 cup strawberries

¼ cup almond milk

1 tsp chia seeds

Directions

Place all ingredients into blender and blend until smooth.

Nutty Banana Smoothie

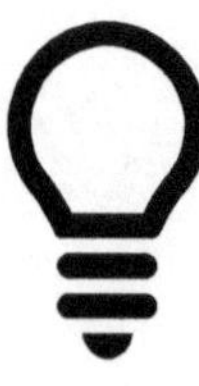

This smoothie targets hair skin and nails and is rich in biotin!

Serves 2

Ingredients

1 ripe banana

6-8 frozen strawberries

5 raw and shelled walnuts

1 cup coconut water

Directions

Place all ingredients into blender and mix until smooth. Garnish with strawberry.

Orange Avocado Smoothie

Targets dry hair and skin!

Serves 2

Ingredients

2 carrots peeled and grated

1 ripe avocado

1 cup vanilla Greek yogurt

Directions

Place all ingredients in blender, mix until smooth. Garnish with carrot shavings

Spinach Cooler

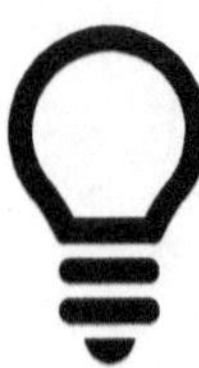

Targets hair, spinach is packed with iron which helps transport oxygen to hair.

Serves 1-2

Ingredients

1 cup frozen spinach

1 tbsp chia seeds

½ banana sliced

½ cup almond milk

½ cup crushed ice

Directions

Place all items in blender, blend until smooth. (place ice closest to your blade.)

Strawberry Apple Smoothie

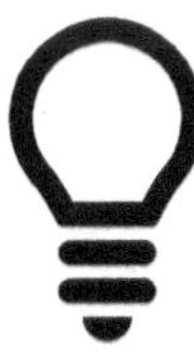

Targets hair growth! This smoothie is rich in beta carotene

Serves 1

Ingredients

1 apple

1 carrot

3-4 strawberries

3-4 cubes of ice

Garnish

1 strawberry

1 tbsp apple granola

1 tsp Greek yogurt

1 tsp organic honey

Directions

Place all ingredients in blender and blend until smooth. Garnish with strawberry, apple granola and drizzle on honey.

**Tip- add a banana if your hair is dry.

Cucumber Cooler

Serves 1

Ingredients

3 carrots

½ cucumber

2 celery sticks, chopped

1 apple sliced

½ cup crushed ice

Directions

Place all ingredients in blender, blend until smooth.

Banana Split Smoothie

Serves 1-2

Ingredients

1 ½ bananas sliced

1 cup pineapple

1 cup vanilla Greek yogurt

1 cup dark frozen sweet cherries

1 cup pineapple coconut waters

1 tsp cacao powder

1 tbsp. almond butter

Directions

Place all ingredients in blender blend until smooth. Garnish with cherry and sprinkle some banana nut granola on top.

Medley Smoothie

Serves 1-2

Ingredients

½ banana

½ sweet potato

1 mandarin orange peeled

½ cup frozen spinach

½ cup pineapple

1 cup pineapple coconut water

Directions

Place all ingredients into blender blend until smooth.

SMOOTHIE BOWLS

Smoothie bowls are exactly what they sound like, it's a smoothie in a bowl. It's an alternative to eating cereal, or drinking a smoothie. Yes, now you can have your smoothie with a spoon. You may need to experiment at first to obtain the right consistency for you. I suggest adding any liquid last so that you can control the thickness of your smoothie. You can also add powders to help thicken and add creaminess to your smoothies. I personally don't use these powders because I like control of every ingredient.

The best part about smoothie bowls is that you can enjoy limitless toppings. Who wouldn't enjoy those?

The next pages include a few of my favorite smoothie bowls recipes, feel free to tweak them to your liking. Don't forget to pile on those toppings to make the most of your smoothie bowl experience. Here are some examples of toppings you may want to try; bananas, sliced apples, pears, kiwis, mango, sliced peaches, strawberries, blueberries, dragon fruit, avocados, chia seeds, nuts, granola etc.

Kale and Avocado Smoothie Bowl

Serves 1

Ingredients

½ Avocado

1 cup baby kale

1 frozen banana sliced

1 cup almond milk

1 tsp organic maple syrup

3-4 cubes of ice

Directions

Blend all ingredients together until smooth but thick enough to spoon. Spoon into bowl top with raspberries and bananas (or what you have on hand). Drizzle on some organic maple syrup.

Oatmeal Cookie Smoothie Bowl

Serves 1

Ingredients

1 Frozen banana

1 cup Oats

½ cup Almond milk

1 tsp flaxseed

1 tsp Vanilla

1 tsp Pumpkin pie spice

1 tsp Almond butter

1 tsp Coconut sugar

 1 tsp Cinnamon

2-3 ice cubes

Directions

Blend all ingredients slowly checking for consistency the texture should be thick enough to spoon. Once blended, slowly add in almond milk stir to desired consistency. Garnish with bananas, granola, fresh strawberries.

Berry Delight Smoothie Bowl

Serves 1

Ingredients

1 ½ cups of frozen mixed berries

1 frozen banana

¼ cup Greek Yogurt (any flavor)

¼ cup pomegranate juice

½ cup sliced peaches

2-3 ice cubes

Directions

Blend all ingredients together until smooth but thick enough to spoon. Transfer into bowl and top with blueberries, sliced peaches and nuts of your choice. Drizzle yogurt over everything

All Green Smoothie Bowl

Serves 1

Ingredients

1 cup spinach

1 cup kale

½ avocado

½ green grapes seedless

1 tablespoon chia seeds

1 frozen banana

½ cup almond milk

3-4 ice cubes

Directions

Blend everything together slowly checking the consistency. Once blended to desired consistency, transfer to bowl. Top with sliced apples, bananas and avocado sprinkle with nuts or granola.

Dragon Fruit Smoothie Bowl

*Author Favorite

Serves 1

Ingredients

1 packet of frozen pitaya puree or 2 dragon fruits (red)

1 cup of frozen pineapple

1 cup of mango

½ kiwi (peeled)

1 handful of spinach

½ cup almond milk

3-4 ice cups to thicken

Directions

Blend all ingredients together until smooth and thick enough to spoon. Top with sliced peaches, bananas, Kiwi. and granola

**If you are unable to find dragon fruit where you live, you can find the puree at https://www.Pitayaplus.com

Blueberry Banana Smoothie Bowl

Serves 1

Ingredients

2 handfuls of spinach

1 frozen banana

1 cup frozen blueberries

1 sliced apple

1 tablespoon organic almond butter (optional)

½ cup almond or coconut milk

1-2 packs of stevia (optional)

Vanilla Greek yogurt (save for topping)

2-3 ice cubes

Directions

Add all ingredients to blender except yogurt, blend until thick and smooth

Cherry Smoothie Bowl

Serves 1

Ingredients

2/3 cups frozen sweet dark cherries

½ cup frozen Raspberries

2 cups cacao powder

1 tsp coconut flakes

½ tbsp. maple syrup

¼ rolled oats

½ cup coconut milk

Directions

Place all items into blender and blend until thick enough to spoon. Pour into your bowl top with fruit and nuts as desired.

Strawberries and Cream Smoothie Bowl

Serves 1

94

Ingredients

1 cup frozen strawberries

1 cup Vanilla Greek Yogurt

1 tsp maple syrup

1 tsp vanilla extract or vanilla flavored stevia liquid

Directions

Blend all ingredients together until thick and smooth.

Toppings

¼ cup cornflakes

¼ cup strawberries

¼ cup blueberries

¼ cup almonds,

¼ cup chia seeds

 Drizzle yogurt over everything

Triple P Smoothie Bowl

Serves 1

Ingredients

1 cup pineapple chunks

1 sliced pear

1 cup frozen peaches

½ cup coconut water

1 tsp honey

Directions

Blend all of the above ingredients together until thick and smooth.

<u>Toppings</u>

¼ cup fresh peaches

¼ cup blackberries

¼ cup granola or your favorite grain cereal

The toppings are peach, blackberries, sunflower seeds, and puffed rice cereal. Get the recipe at the bottom of the post.

Kiwi Kale Smoothie Bowl

Serves 1

Ingredients

1 handful of baby kale

I kiwi sliced

1 banana sliced

1 cup avocado

1 cup almond milk

2-3 ice cubes

Directions

Blend all the above ingredients together until thick and smooth, slowly pour milk in until you reach desired consistency to spoon.

<u>Toppings</u>

¼ cup raspberries

½ sliced banana

1 sliced kiwi

¼ chia seeds

Place fruit in rows on top of smoothie mix.

Almond Butter and Raspberry Smoothie Cup

Serves 1

INGREDIENTS

1 large banana
1 cup raspberries
½ cup almond milk
2-3 cubes of ice
2 Tbsp. almond butter
1 Tbsp. honey

¼ cup vanilla yogourt

PREPARATION

Blend the banana, raspberries, almond milk, ice, almond butter, and 1 tablespoon of the honey until smooth.

Toppings

¼ cup Strawberries

¼ coconut flakes

 ¼ cup raspberries

¼ cup granola

Drizzle maple syrup on top

Serve in dessert cup.

Orange Berry Smoothie Bowl

Serves 1

INGREDIENTS

1 banana

1 cup of blueberries, blackberries
½ cup orange juice

2-3 cubes of ice

PREPARATION

Blend the banana, berries, ice and orange juice until smooth. Transfer to a bowl and add toppings.

Toppings

¼ blackberries, blueberries, and walnuts

Mixed Berry Smoothie Bowl

Serves 1

INGREDIENTS

1 ½ cups frozen mixed berries (such as strawberries, raspberries, and blueberries)
¼ cup pomegranate juice
¼ cup plain yogurt, plus additional for drizzling
½ cup blueberries
½ peach, sliced
2 Tbsp. dried mulberries
2 Tbsp. pumpkin seeds

PREPARATION

Blend the frozen berries, pomegranate juice, and ¼ cup of the yogurt until smooth. Transfer to a bowl or tall cup and top with the blueberries, peach, mulberries, pumpkin seeds, and a drizzle of yogurt.

Chocolate Peanut Butter and Banana Smoothie Bowl

Serves 1

INGREDIENTS

1 cup almond milk
1 large banana, sliced
1 cup ice
2 Tbsp. peanut butter
1 Tbsp. unsweetened cocoa powder
¼ tsp pure vanilla extract
1 Tbsp. maple syrup
2 Tbsp. cocoa nibs
2 Tbsp. granola
2 Tbsp. chopped peanuts

PREPARATION

Blend the almond milk, ½ the banana, ice, peanut butter, cocoa powder, vanilla extract, and maple syrup until smooth. Transfer to a bowl and top with the cocoa nibs, granola, chopped peanuts, and remaining ½ banana.

Blueberry, Spinach, and Pineapple Smoothie Bowl

Serves 1

INGREDIENTS

1 cup baby spinach leaves
1 ½ cups blueberries
½ cup apple juice
½ cup ice
½ cup chopped pineapple
¼ cup puffed rice cereal, such as Rice Krispies.
2 Tbsp. pumpkin seeds
1 Tbsp. flax seeds
Honey, for drizzling

Directions

Blend the spinach, 1 cup of the blueberries, apple juice, and ice until smooth. Transfer to a bowl and top with the pineapple, puffed rice, pumpkin seeds, flax seeds, remaining ½ cup blueberries, and a drizzle of honey.

Sweet Potato Pie Smoothie Bowl

Serves 1

INGREDIENTS

1 large banana
½ cup frozen sweet potato
¼ tsp pure vanilla extract
¼ tsp ground cinnamon,

¼ cup walnuts
2 Tbsp. shredded coconut

PREPARATION

Blend the banana, carrot juice, ice, 2 of the dates, vanilla, and cinnamon until smooth. Transfer to a bowl and top with the walnuts, coconut, remaining 2 dates, and a dusting of cinnamon.

Banana Nut Oats and Smoothie Bowl

Serves 1

Ingredients

1 sliced banana

2 tsp flaxseeds

1 cup oats

1 cup almond milk

½ cup almonds

Toppings

¼ cup coconut flakes

¼ cup granola

3 sliced strawberries

1 sliced banana

A few berries

Directions

Place all ingredients in blender except topping blend able to spoon Pour into bowl and add toppings.

DETOX WATER

Detox waters are a great way to lose weight and detox your body quickly and effectively. Detoxing is one of the best ways to rid your body of harmful toxins. The body needs at least 6-8, 8-ounce glasses of water a day, however your personal daily amount can differ from person to person.

This detox section will provide you with a few refreshing and tasty recipes to detox yourself and increase your water intake daily. I have provided a detailed ingredient list at the beginning of this book, please refer to that list to help you create the most beneficial detox water for your personal needs. Feel free to play around with fruits and flavors that are appealing to your taste buds. The recipes in this section are some of the most common detox water recipes that many have used and obtained desired results. You will see an immediate difference in your energy levels, appetite, and overall skin appearance.

The amount of time you decide to detox will depend on your individual needs and goals. Some people do a cleanse and detox over a 3-day period, while others detox for a week, 30 days and sometimes longer. It is always a good rule of thumb to consult with your doctor before detoxing. To get the best results while detoxing you may want to avoid high fructose drinks, sodas, processed foods and refined sugars.

Lemon Cucumber Mint Detox

Serves 1

Ingredients

2 lemons sliced

1 cucumber sliced skin on

8 organic mint leaves

4 Tbsp., Braggs apple cider vinegar

1 gallon of water (spring, distilled or filtered)

Instructions:

1.Wash and dry lemons and cucumbers then slice.

2. Place all fruit and mint in bottom of pitcher.

3. Fill with water and shake.

4. Refrigerate for 12 hours to allow infusion and enjoy.

Lemon Berry Detox

Serves 1

Ingredients

2 sliced lemons

½ cup raspberries

½ cup strawberries

½ cup blueberries

1 gallon of water (distilled, filtered or spring)

Directions

Place all fruit in bottom of pitcher, add water, shake. Refrigerate for 12 hours and enjoy!

Cucumber Watermelon Mint Detox

Serves 1

Ingredients

1 cup pureed watermelon (seedless)

1 cucumber sliced

8 organic mint leaves

1-gallon water (spring, filtered or distilled)

Directions

Place cucumbers, watermelon, and mint leaves in pitcher. Fill pitcher with water, shake well. Refrigerate for 12 hours shake and enjoy.

Orange Detox

Serves 1

Ingredients

2 navel oranges sliced

8 organic mint leaves

1 lime sliced

1 gallon of water (spring, filtered or distilled)

Directions

Wash and slice all fruit, then place in bottom of pitcher with mint leaves.

Shake refrigerate and enjoy.

Lemon Lime Mint Detox

Serves 1

Ingredients

2 sliced limes

2 sliced lemons

8 organic mint leaves

1 gallon (spring, distilled or filtered water)

Directions

Place all fruit in bottom of pitcher, add water. Refrigerate for 12 hours and enjoy.

Kiwi Peach Mint Raspberry

Serves 1

Ingredients

1 kiwi sliced

1 peach sliced

8 organic mint leaves

1 gallon of water (spring, filtered or distilled

Directions

Wash and slice all fruit place in pitcher with mint leaves add water. Refrigerate for 12 hours and enjoy.

Blueberry Orange Mint Detox

Serves 1

Ingredients

1 navel orange

1 cup blueberries

8 mint leaves

1 gallon filtered or spring water

Directions

Place fruit and mint leaves in bottom of pitcher and fill with filtered water. Chill overnight and enjoy.

Strawberry Lemon Basil Mint Detox

Serves 1

112

Ingredients

1 cup fresh strawberries washed

2 lemons washed and sliced

6 8 basil leaves

1 cucumber sliced and washed

1 cup organic lemon juice

1/2 tsp cayenne pepper

1-gallon spring or filtered water

Directions

Place fruit and basil leaves in pitcher then add cayenne pepper and lemon juice. Fill with spring or filtered water.

Citrus Detox Water

Serves 1

113

Ingredients

1 grapefruit

1 navel orange

1 lemon

1 tsp honey

Directions

Slice all fruit place in bottom of pitcher fill with water and chill overnight.

Pineapple Lime Detox Water

Serves 1

Ingredients

2 whole limes

1 cup sliced pineapple wedges

2 parsley leaves

1 gallon of spring or filtered water

Directions

Squeeze fresh juice from both limes into pitcher, add lemon wedges, pineapple wedges and parsley. Fill pitcher with water and chill for 12 hours. Enjoy.

Minty Strawberry Lemon Lime Water

Serves 1

115

Ingredients

½ cup strawberry puree

1 lemon sliced

1 lime sliced

1 cup strawberries

8 mint leaves

1-gallon spring or filtered water

Directions

place all food and mint leaves in in pitcher, fill with water. Let sit overnight. Shake or stir before use.

30 Day Detox Water Challenge

Serves 1

Ingredients

2 organic lemons washed and sliced

2 organic limes washed and sliced

2 tsp Bragg organic apple cider vinegar with the Mother per 8 oz

2 tsp organic honey

2 tsp cayenne pepper or ground cinnamon

1-gallon Spring or filtered water

**add an orange if too bitter for your taste

Directions

Place lemon and limes in bottom of pitcher, then add remaining ingredients. Let sit in refrigerator overnight. Shake well before each use. I prefer to add ACV per glass than into pitcher with ingredients.

Drink at least 1 gallon a day for 30 days Avoid sodas and sugary drinks, add an exercise routine for optimal results.

Keep in mind that as your body rids itself of toxins, increased bathroom usage is normal.

Grocery List

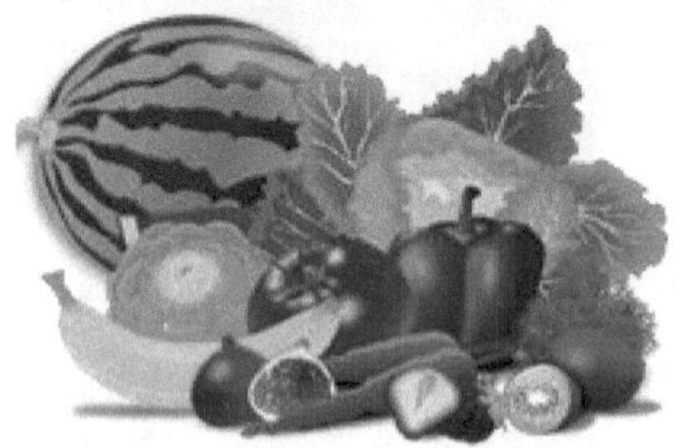

Here is a handy list to get you started Take this with you to the grocery store or use to check off items for your favorite recipes

Apples	Coconut oil	Mint leaves
Apple Cider Vinegar	Coconut water-	Mustard greens
Avocado	Dragon fruit	Oranges
Bananas	Greek yogurt	Pineapple
Blueberries	Granola	Pineapple juice
Carrots	Guava	Raspberries-
Cherries	Guava juice-	Romaine lettuce-
Chia Seeds	Honey organic-	Spinach
Cinnamon	Kale	Strawberries.
Cinnamon sticks	Lemons	Sweet Potato-frozen/canned
Cucumber	Lemon juice	Squash
Coconut flakes	Melons	watermelon

Goals:____

____

____

____

____

____

____

____

____

____

____

____

____

____

____

____

____

____

____

30 DAY DETOX CHALLENGE

Starting weight__________

Ending Weight__________

Starting Date____________

End date________________

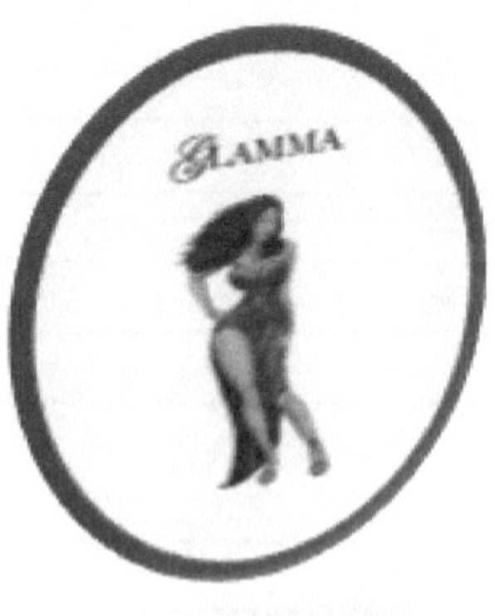

Other books from Author Zena Xenae

Available on Amazon.com, Barnes and Noble, Createspace, and your local bookstore.

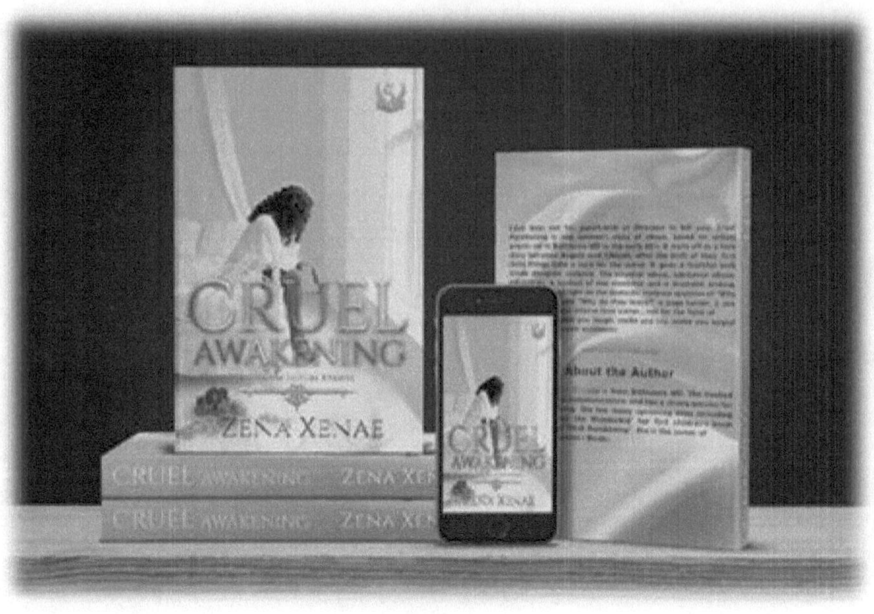

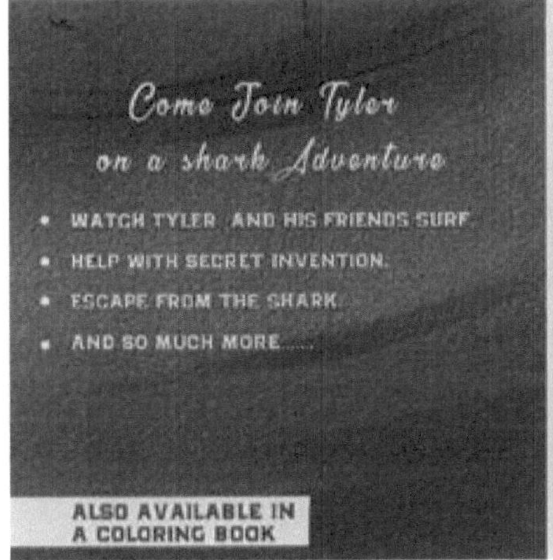

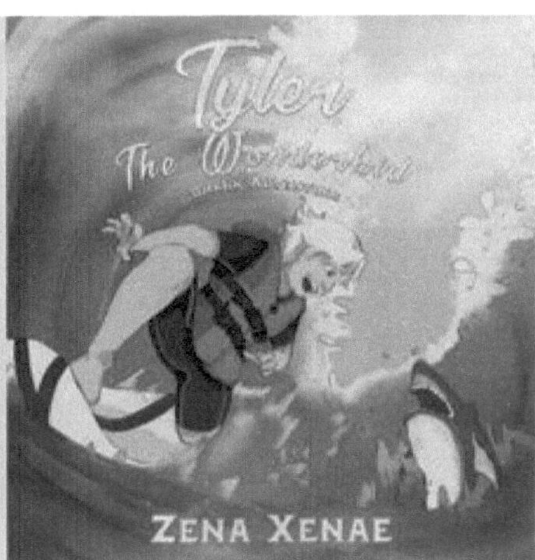

Follow us to stay updated!

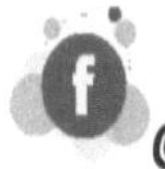 **@cruelawakening the book**

IG:cruelawakening

Live demos on YT subscribe to Zena Xenae

Email us: glammabooks@gmail.com

COMING FALL OF 2018

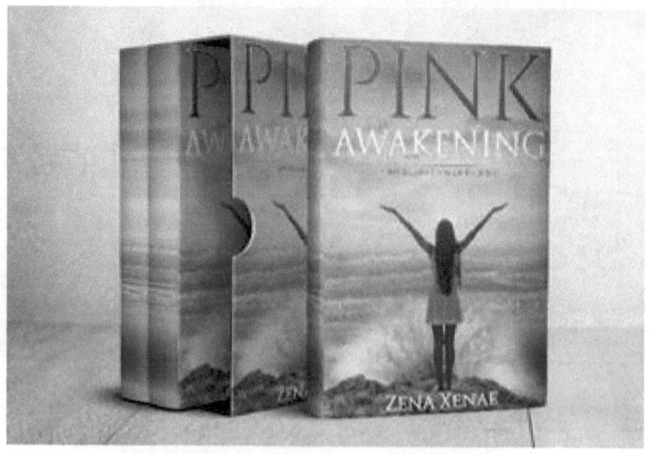

A MEMIOR ABOUT SURVIVAL

Coming Soon......Pink Awakening, Chemo Curls, Bert's Porch, How to Survive Student Loans, Blue Awakening .